The Career Development Framework:
Guiding Principles for Occupational Therapy

Implementation guide

Royal College of Occupational Therapists

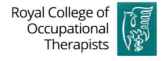

First published in 2017
by the Royal College of Occupational Therapists Ltd
106–114 Borough High Street, London SE1 1LB
www.rcot.org.uk

Copyright © Royal College of Occupational Therapists 2017

Authors: Royal College of Occupational Therapists
Writers: Dr Stephanie Tempest, Dr Karina Dancza
Date for review: 2019

This information may be reproduced and adapted for personal/professional use by occupational therapy personnel. Where using and/or adapting this work, please acknowledge the Royal College of Occupational Therapists as publishers of the original edition, and contact us with details of how you intend to use the information to help us to evaluate the uptake and impact of the resource. Permission for other uses including, but not limited to, the use by organisations and professions beyond occupational therapy, translation, multiple copying, use within new published works and resale, should be requested from the Publications Manager at the Royal College of Occupational Therapists. Before seeking permission, please check our open permissions licence (**https://www.rcot.co.uk/practice-resources/rcot-publications/copying-and-permissions**) and the terms of any applicable licences e.g. from the Copyright Licensing Agency, to see if these meet your needs.

Other enquiries about this document should be addressed to the Education and Research Team at the Royal College of Occupational Therapists at eda@rcot.co.uk or at the above address.

British Library cataloguing in publication data
A catalogue record for this book is available from the British Library

ISBN 978-1-905944-67-5

Whilst every effort is made to ensure accuracy, the Royal College of Occupational Therapists shall not be liable for any loss or damage either directly or indirectly resulting from the use of this publication.

Typeset by Fish Books Ltd

Digitally printed on demand in Great Britain by the Lavenham Press, Suffolk

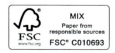

Contents

1   **Introducing the Career Development Framework**   1
      What is it?   1
      What isn't it?   2
      How can the Career Framework be used?   4
      What about specific competency frameworks?   6
      What else do I need?   6

2   **Examples from the profession**   7
      Bringing the Career Development Framework to life   7

      Sandra M. Rowan (occupational therapist, independent practitioner)   8

      Donna Malley (occupational therapist, National Health Service)   12

      Christine Craik (occupational therapist, independent consultant, Editor-in-Chief *British Journal of Occupational Therapy*)   18

      Amanda Sullivan (student and social care support worker)   23

      Dr Patricia McClure (occupational therapist, academic, Chair of Council RCOT)   28

Contents

3 What next — **34**
   Further reading — 34
   Top tips for using the Career Framework — 35

Acknowledgements   **Inside back cover**

1 Introducing the Career Development Framework

What is it?

Welcome to the implementation guide for the *Career Development Framework: guiding principles for occupational therapy*. This guide is designed to offer ideas and tips for using the Career Development Framework (also referred to here as the Career Framework). The detailed Career Development Framework is open access for all and available at *www.rcot.co.uk*. RCOT members can also find tools to support them when using the Career Framework in practice, via the members' pages on the website.

The Career Framework is an overarching set of guiding principles for occupational therapy and offers a structured process to guide careers, learning and development within the occupational therapy profession. It contains four interacting Pillars of Practice (Professional Practice; Facilitation of Learning; Leadership; and Evidence, Research and Development), each with nine Levels.

Introducing the Career Development Framework

What isn't it?

The resource is not about pay, terms and conditions or your current job level, band or grade. It is not a performance management tool. Neither is it a competency framework. This Career Framework provides a set of guiding principles; it is all about you and your development. It can help you identify the skills, knowledge and mind-set you already have or those you wish to develop, regardless of your setting or area of practice. It is a Career Framework for all of us.

The Career Framework Pillars of Practice

Professional Practice	Maintain occupation at the centre of practice.
	Deliver safe, effective, person-centred and ethical practice.
	Use of professional judgement, reasoning and decision making.
Facilitation of Learning	Teach, mentor, supervise and/or assess others.
	Facilitate placement learning.
	Create and evaluate learning environments, tools and materials.
Leadership	Identify, monitor and enhance own knowledge and skills.
	Guide, direct and/or facilitate teamwork.
	Design, implement and manage professional and/or organisational change.
Evidence, Research and Development	Influence broader socio-economic and political agendas.
	Create, use and/or translate evidence to inform practice.
	Design, implement, evaluate and disseminate research.

Career Development Framework: implementation guide

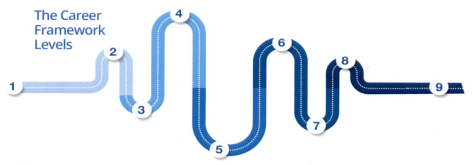

The Career Framework Levels

① Level 1
basic general knowledge and an awareness of the role of occupational therapy

entry level; undertakes a limited number of straightforward tasks under direct supervision; any new starter to work in the sector, not necessarily straight from school; may progress rapidly to Level 2; aware of service improvement projects, and the need for self-development

② Level 2
basic understanding of occupational therapy and the field of work

may carry out practice based, technical, scientific or administrative duties per established protocols or procedures, with guidance and supervision; participates in service improvement; beginning to identify areas for self-development

③ Level 3
knowledge and understanding of occupational therapy procedures, processes and general concepts in a field of work

may carry out a wide range of delegated duties with guidance and supervision available when needed; contributes to service improvement, and is responsible for self-development

④ Level 4
knowledge and understanding of occupational therapy principles, procedures, processes and general concepts within a field of work

guided by standard operating procedures and protocols; makes judgements, plans activities; contributes to service improvement and demonstrates self-development; may have responsibility for aspects of supervision of some staff or students

⑤ Level 5
comprehensive, specialised, factual and theoretical knowledge and understanding of occupational therapy and of the boundaries of that knowledge

creative problem-solver; makes judgements within own scope of work; actively contributes to service improvement and self-development; may have responsibility for supervision of staff or students; may be eligible for registration with the Health and Care Professions Council (the regulatory body in the United Kingdom) as an occupational therapist, or may be non-regulated and have own specialist trade or craft e.g. posture and seating skills

⑥ Level 6
critical understanding of theory and practical occupational therapy knowledge

leads in a specific area with some responsibility for service and team performance; creative problem-solver; supervises staff / students; consistently undertakes self-development

⑦ Level 7
highly specialised knowledge and critical awareness

Specialist practice-based, technical or scientific skills; innovative; responsible for service development in complex environments; leads within services/research/education contexts; supervises staff/students; pro-actively self-develops

⑧ Level 8
most advanced and specialised knowledge

at the forefront of the profession; strategic leader; political influencer; original thinker; responsible for finances, service development and/or multiple teams; supervises staff/students; intuitively self-develops

⑨ Level 9
innovate and advance occupational therapy in the wider context

develops services to a population; works at the highest level of an organisation; accountable for the performance of staff/services; thinks at a systems level; supervises staff/students; intuitively self-develops

How can the Career Framework be used?

As an occupational therapist, support worker, student or someone who is interested in developing a career in occupational therapy, you can:

- Map your current skills and experience into the Pillars at various Levels to highlight your abilities, preferably with a critical and trusted friend or colleague.

- Identify and plan the learning opportunities you need to support your professional development, e.g. when preparing for mentoring, supervision or appraisal.

- Rely on the Career Framework to maintain your occupational therapy identity when working in generic roles or diverse settings.

- Use the principles to articulate your transferable skills when planning a move between different settings (and/or different countries), e.g. into research, practice, academia, leadership or emerging roles.

- Articulate your lifelong career pathway within the profession.

As a person who accesses occupational therapy services, you can:

- Be reassured that the Career Framework places expectations in terms of knowledge, skills and ways of thinking for the occupational therapy personnel you work with.

As an employer or manager, you can:

- Use the Career Framework in the development of job descriptions.
- Understand the learning and development needs of individuals or groups in appraisals/supervision including '360 degree' reviews.
- Support staff retention and the most appropriate skill mix within a setting.

As a funder or commissioner of services, you can:

- Use the Career Framework to help understand the broad knowledge and skills that occupational therapy personnel can offer.
- Support the most effective and efficient use of occupational therapy personnel within and across services.

For the profession, we can:

- Reinforce an occupation-centred identity as the unique selling point of the profession, regardless of setting.
- Emphasise the range of knowledge and skills across the four Pillars of Practice.
- Give prominence to our unique and pivotal role within teams.
- Identify experts across the four Pillars to nurture and make full use of occupational therapy talent.
- Articulate our right to apply for non-occupational therapy specific roles and / or promote the introduction of new occupational therapy roles in diverse settings.

What about specific competency frameworks?

If you are seeking to develop local, context-specific competencies, you can still use the Career Framework, but will need to do so alongside national occupational standards, e.g. UK National Occupational Standards (NOS: *http://www.ukstandards.org.uk/Pages/index.aspx*).

What else do I need?

You need to access the main Career Framework which is available at *www.rcot.co.uk* and contains all the guiding principles for each Pillar and Level. The Career Framework is also intended to be used alongside other key documents including The Royal College of Occupational Therapists' *Code of ethics and professional conduct*, the *Professional standards*, the *Learning and development standards for pre-registration education* and standards from the Health and Care Professions Council.

Several key documents were reviewed and incorporated into this Career Framework. These are highlighted in Appendix 1 of the main document. It is anticipated that within local areas or specialisms, other frameworks will need to be aligned. The Career Framework offers the guiding principles to facilitate this process and enable transferability of occupational therapy careers across areas and sectors.

2 Examples from the profession

Bringing the Career Development Framework to life

Grateful thanks to Sandra, Donna, Christine, Amanda and Patricia who gave their time so freely and shared their own thoughts on the Career Framework. While acknowledging that it is difficult to capture the true breadth and diversity of people and settings in our profession within five case studies alone, these should help bring to life the opportunities presented by the resource for everyone.

Sandra M. Rowan
Occupational therapist, independent practitioner   8

Donna Malley
Occupational therapist, National Health Service   12

Christine Craik
Occupational therapist, independent consultant,
Editor-in-Chief *British Journal of Occupational Therapy*   18

Amanda Sullivan
Student and social care support worker   23

Dr Patricia McClure
Occupational therapist, academic, Chair of Council RCOT   28

Sandra M. Rowan

MA Dip COT

Consultant in Workforce Development

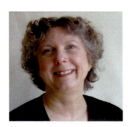

Profile as mapped to the Career Framework:	
■ Professional Practice	6
■ Facilitation of Learning	8
■ Leadership	8
■ Evidence, Research and Development	7

Background

I am a proud occupational therapist. I have worked in many roles within the National Health Service, academia and independent practice. No matter what I do or where I go, I always promote myself as an occupational therapist. My current work as an independent practitioner is focused on workforce development across all professions in the health sector, as an associate with Skills for Health and as a supervisor for senior allied health professionals. Previously I have worked in academia, lecturing, placement co-ordination and student coaching/mentoring. I have also worked as a clinician across primary, secondary and community care with a special interest in neurology, oncology and palliative care. I gained management experience at operational and strategic levels in National Health Service trusts and at a strategic health authority.

My career profile

I really liked that you can be at various levels for different Pillars. Wherever I think I am today, I know that it will be different from where I will be in 6–12 months' time. For me, shifts in where I place myself depend on what my focus has been and the opportunities I have had.

Looking at my own career profile now, I placed myself comfortably in Level 8 for Leadership and Facilitation of Learning, as my current role demands these skills of me. At times, I may even place myself at Level 9. In contrast, I am not currently working as a practitioner, so I think I am at Level 6 for Professional Practice. For me that means that I would need to brush up on my skills should I decide to take on a professional practice role. Similarly, for Evidence, Research and Development, I see myself at Level 7. I am a consumer of research. I use evidence to inform and critique my practice, but I am not a researcher and I am OK with that for now.

How I use the Career Framework

For all the statements, I asked myself "what does this mean to me?" The Career Framework cannot define all areas of practice. I know I need to define what it looks like in my situation and consider how I meet a specific statement.

There is no doubt that the statements in the Career Framework can be quite challenging. I use the descriptors as a trigger point to reflect on my own development. Sometimes I am surprised as perhaps I am up a level because I have learnt something new in the past year. Other times I feel I have slipped back as I have decided to focus elsewhere. I am comfortable with that, but it can make you feel exposed.

I believe challenging ourselves is so important because we need to keep developing our practice. People we work for have a right to know that we are at the top of our game. It can be a scary experience; but questioning ourselves is healthy as it can prompt us to find out more.

The Career Framework is different from Agenda for Change used within the National Health Service. Agenda for Change is about pay and conditions. The Career Framework is about knowledge, skills, understanding, development and progression; it is about what you look like in your practice and how you behave. It is not just about a qualification, it is about how you think, reflect and change your practice.

Learning and development is a key part of being a professional. That is where the Career Framework comes into play. It is not about money or climbing the ladder; it is about doing the best job you can at the point you are. If you have been in a job for a while, it can be tough to look for opportunities to develop. The Career Framework makes you look at your own practice. It makes me feel in control of my career.

Being an independent practitioner

As an independent practitioner, it is sometimes tricky to consider where I am in my career. I don't have the structures of an established institution and a hierarchy to map myself against. I see the Career Framework helping me with this. It can also identify where I might need to access further support.

I don't read the descriptors literally; I re-interpret them to fit my world. I see the Career Framework statements as written in a way which are intended to be interpreted and reshaped. Does it matter that all statements don't fit? I don't think so. Is this statement absolutely essential to me being able to perform in this Pillar? If yes, find a way to include it. If not, then move on.

Take-home message

I think the Career Framework and the Pillars help you to think about your own career. It is important to remember that the Pillars all interlink and shift at different points in your working life. I can see the Career Framework as a useful structure which encourages you to step back and look at where you are and where you would like to be, so you can seek out opportunities for further professional development.

Donna Malley

Dip. COT, BSc Hons Health Studies,
MSt Primary and Community Care

Occupational Therapy Clinical Specialist –
Oliver Zangwill Centre for Neuropsychological Rehabilitation

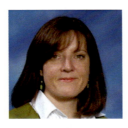

Profile as mapped to the Career Framework:	
■ Professional Practice	8
■ Facilitation of Learning	7
■ Leadership	7
■ Evidence, Research and Development	6

Background

I have worked as an occupational therapist for the past 30 years, including over 20 years specialising with adults with acquired brain injury. I joined the team at the Oliver Zangwill Centre for Neuropsychological Rehabilitation in 1998, where I achieved my MSt in Primary and Community Care. Since then I have also undertaken a Quality Improvement Fellowship, NIHR CLAHRC Fellowship and participated in secondment opportunities to enhance my professional skills and experience. I am passionate about supporting the profession through engagement as chair of the Royal College of Occupational Therapists Specialist Section – Neurological Practice, Brain Injury Forum committee, and co-editing guidelines for occupational therapists working with adults with acquired brain injury (2013).

My career profile

Having been in the National Health Service all my career, my first thought when looking at the Career Framework was, "does my Agenda for Change pay banding map onto these levels?". It quickly became apparent, however, that I was not consistently on a single Level for all Pillars, so that made me rethink how I was going to use this document!

I believe it is brave and necessary for the profession to encompass the four Pillars as vital elements of our practice. This does not mean it is a straightforward process in terms of matching one's skills to Levels within these Pillars. Even though I have done a masters degree and I have had the opportunity to be involved in research activities with people who are leaders in research, I felt that I was much stronger in the Professional Practice Pillar than I was in the other Pillars. It was interesting to do the Career Framework as a self-reflective exercise on my own, however I would be interested to know if I sat down with someone who knows me well, would my Levels change in response to their reflections?

Am I placing myself on the right level?

I use reflection a lot in my work and I am comfortable being a reflective practitioner. Even with this, I still found myself questioning if I was 'advanced' or 'most advanced' in my practice. I think it is quite common for us to believe that others must know more than you do!

Examples from the profession

I placed myself at Level 8 in Professional Practice, but I acknowledge I did this for my current clinical role. I consider I have specific knowledge, skills and competencies through working for many years in this specialist field. If I moved into another area of occupational therapy practice, I would drop back on Levels of some Pillars straight away. However, I would like to think that I could move up the Levels again using my transferable knowledge, but acknowledge that this would take time.

Over the years I have discovered that the more you think you know the more you realise you don't know! You have transferable skills, but you have to acknowledge your boundaries in terms of your scope of practice and you have a lot to learn. I think the Career Framework could help you understand that transition.

If people want examples of what is different between say, Levels 8 and 9 in a specialism, I think it would be difficult to have a blanket list. So, while it may not suit everyone to have the Career Framework this flexible, I think it is the discussion this stimulates which is the important focus. We need to negotiate what it means to be at a Level 9; this leaves open the possibility to strive for more.

The Career Framework has made me think of getting people together within my team to see where we place ourselves and what we might need to do to progress our service.

Don't see the Pillars separately!

The Pillars are not mutually exclusive. There isn't much duplication between the Pillars, which means that you can't just pull out one Pillar and map yourself onto that (for example pulling out only the Professional Practice Pillar if you are in a health role, or Evidence, Research and Development Pillar if you are in an academic researcher role).

There are, however, elements of each Pillar within **all areas of work**. That is a crucial point. I have heard people say, "I don't do research", and the danger is that they do not see evidence, research and development as important in their role. But by having the four Pillars of Practice in the Career Framework we can articulate how all roles have elements of each Pillar.

Using the Career Framework in a team

The Career Framework is a great reflective tool; I can't praise it enough. It gives you a language to help you make sense of all the elements within your role and it makes you stop, think and challenge your perceptions of what you think you know. This I believe has utility not only for individuals, but also for teams, e.g. for service design and improvements.

The Career Framework could be useful to help articulate some of the competing demands or expectations within a job role. I think there is often an unhelpful separation between academia and practice, summarised in the phrase "theory-practice gap". When services prioritise clinical productivity, often aspects such as research become sidelined. If teams can share the skills within their service across the four Pillars, it might help us to highlight where we could target and develop our services further.

It made me think about how we could use the Career Framework to map our service, so that team members are encouraged to discuss where they feel the team is functioning. This could create interesting conversations about how the team could develop and it would not be quite so exposing for individuals and reliant on them sharing their own Levels.

The information generated from these team discussions could inform our Continuing Professional Development (CPD) provision. We could map where we would like development and link it with the available offer. We could also target our own courses to specific Pillars and Levels, supporting those accessing our courses to select appropriate opportunities. I think the Career Framework would help us as a service to 'join the dots' between our skills, service delivery and the CPD needs and provision.

I haven't seen another document demonstrate the skills we have across the four Pillars so comprehensively, yet succinctly. Using the Career Framework at a strategic level is going to be transformational.

Take-home message

People will need to think about the Career Framework for themselves in their own context; it is not for the Royal College to tell us what 'specialist' looks like. It invites and creates curiosity. What people will learn and benefit from are the debates and discussions we will have. It comes alive when you talk about it and I would encourage everyone to get talking! Spark ideas off about where services define themselves and how it is used. It is going to be really exciting to see where it heads in the future. I think it will have more spin-offs than we can think about right now.

My suggestion is to keep track of what you are doing with the Career Framework so we can see how it progresses. Lightbulb moments are fleeting so we need to capture and share these for the benefit of our profession.

Christine Craik

OBE, MPhil, FRCOT, DMS, MCMI, FHEA

Independent Consultant and Editor-in-Chief
British Journal of Occupational Therapy

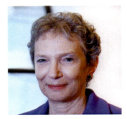

Profile as mapped to the Career Framework:	
■ Professional Practice	7
■ Facilitation of Learning	9
■ Leadership	9
■ Evidence, Research and Development	9

Background

I have had a long, diverse and interesting career in occupational therapy. I was formerly a manager of mental health occupational therapy services, before becoming Director of Occupational Therapy at Brunel University London, where I was an academic for 15 years. I was honoured to be appointed OBE for my services to occupational therapy, particularly in relation to mental health and education, having spent much of my clinical career working in, developing and researching mental health services. Since 2014 I have been Editor-In-Chief of the *British Journal of Occupational Therapy*.

My career profile

The most interesting aspect of considering my Career Framework Levels was reflecting on my entire career. I've moved between health services and academic roles several times. To make these transitions, I needed to think about translating my knowledge, skills and expertise into different fields. I can see how the Career Framework, and specifically the four Pillars, could have supported me to make these connections.

I am happy to share where I think I am on the Pillars, although others may not agree. The Career Framework certainly does help stimulate reflection and discussion.

I rated myself at Level 7 for Professional Practice because it has been more than 20 years since I worked clinically. I can also see, however, that I am using my 'professional practice' skills in my managerial and academic roles. For example, I am using specialist communication skills all the time.

In the Facilitation of Learning and Leadership Pillars, I placed myself at Level 9, having done most of what was listed on those Pillars in my previous roles. Although I cannot say that I did everything. I see the Career Framework as more flexible, rather than needing to tick off each statement.

In the Evidence, Research and Development Pillar I began by comparing myself with others. Although I am not a professor of occupational therapy and I have not managed multi-million pound research grants, the research I have done and my involvement with the *British Journal of Occupational Therapy* does, I think, put me at this Level.

I must say that the phrase using the 'most advanced and specialist skills' can be a bit off-putting. I questioned how would I know I am doing that? While it is a challenge to think about what that might look like, it can form a basis for a discussion and it allows for continued growth no matter where you are in your career.

The importance of all four Pillars

The Career Framework highlights various aspects to the profession in the four Pillars. Historically, occupational therapy has focused on the Professional Practice Pillar, as this is the basis of our profession. While this is important, I believe that all four Pillars are required for the roles we do. It might be interesting for people to think about their role in relation to the four Pillars and consider where they have prioritised their skills and where future development is required.

I guess one of the differences I have had in my career is that I moved between health service and academic roles. If I had stayed in one place, I could have developed further in one Pillar, although I think it might have been at the expense of another Pillar. These are the choices we make; to be highly advanced in one area, or have a broad career profile. There are advantages and disadvantages to both.

In the future, we may see a shift in the career profiles of some occupational therapists, where they move earlier into research, leadership or educational roles. This may not be for everyone but we need to value all aspects of the profession. I believe the Career Framework is a way of highlighting the legitimacy of different career pathways in the profession.

The Career Framework supporting career transitions

With occupational therapy moving into increasingly diverse areas, people are likely to have a more varied career path than we have historically seen. I think that occupational therapists will need to convince new employers of their skills and the Career Framework could help facilitate those discussions.

The Career Framework clearly recognises occupation as our unique perspective: that is what we are about. So, we could use the Career Framework to explain our role in a multidisciplinary team.

The Career Framework provides a language to help people articulate their skills through seeing what they are currently doing or have the potential to do, and how this relates to occupational therapy. It can support occupational therapy personnel when they have a career break or transition into another area or into retirement. I think there is a huge, untapped potential in retired occupational therapists and the Career Framework could help match the skills of a person with the available opportunities.

Using the Career Framework for early career planning

Including Levels 1–9 in the Career Framework can help people see possible career pathways for themselves, even before they apply to a university programme. With changes in health, education and social care systems, I believe we need to continue to promote the profession not only to potential new employers, but also people interested in becoming occupational therapists.

The Career Framework can support occupational therapy students in their career planning. It can help them apply their previous learning and skills in an occupational therapy framework. It may also be useful in curriculum design by considering the range of learning opportunities available to students across the four Pillars.

Take-home message

The Career Framework has many possible uses which will only become apparent as we engage with the resource. The key is to use it flexibly. I think its most valuable attribute will be evident as we move to more diverse settings. It has the potential to demonstrate what we have achieved and what we hope to do for a wide range of employers and service users. It is important to move towards an inclusive Career Framework which is not dependent on one setting, so that we can facilitate smooth transitions for occupational therapy personnel between distinct roles.

Amanda Sullivan

Diploma Early Years Education

Occupational Therapy Social Work Assistant and Student

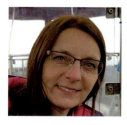

Profile as mapped to the Career Framework:
- Professional Practice — 6
- Facilitation of Learning — 3
- Leadership — 4
- Evidence, Research and Development — 2

Background

I have taken the long way around to find occupational therapy as a career. I initially trained and worked as nursery teacher before trying out social work and completing two years of that degree. I found these careers weren't the right fit for me, so I kept looking. I now work in a social work assistant role in adult and community social care services. Although my job title is social work, I am working as an occupational therapy assistant. Alongside this I am studying part-time for the Agored Cymru Level 3 Diploma in Occupational Therapy Support, which consists of ten core modules related to occupational therapy philosophy and practice. I think I have found the career for me!

My career profile

The Career Framework made me reflect on my skills. I initially read over the statements a few

Examples from the profession

times to consider how they applied to me. I had a go by reading from the top (Level 9) and working backwards, eliminating each part until I saw my own practice. I then sat down and had a conversation with my manager. That was interesting because people see you differently. She knows me well and understands my reasoning and she put me higher than I put myself.

Professional Practice was my strongest Pillar (Level 6), as that has been the focus of my career in this and previous roles. I initially wasn't sure about my Level, but after a discussion with my manager, she confirmed that she also thought I was at Level 6. I don't know if I am at the 'right' level for being a support worker, but for me personally, my previous experiences which I bring to this role mean that I can justify being at that Level.

My other Pillars are less well developed and when I was on the edge, I chose to put myself down a Level so I could feel confident that I could justify how I met each element. I put myself at Level 4 for Leadership and Level 3 for Facilitation of Learning. My lowest Pillar is Evidence, Research and Development (Level 2). I have undertaken research in my previous university courses and I always try to use as much evidence as I can before I make any decisions, but I am not confident with it. Once I have completed my current course, I think I might move up in this Pillar. Getting back into studying has already boosted my confidence.

Using the Career Framework as a support worker

We don't have a job title which relates to occupational therapy (we are social work assistants), so it is hard to gauge where we should be. There is no expectation in the Career Framework that a support worker should be at a certain Level in each Pillar. I like that; it allows me to show I am at various Levels due to my experience. This reflects how you might have a slightly different profile of skills to someone else doing the same job.

Initially I didn't realise that this Career Framework was for everyone, not just for support workers. Because it starts at Level 1 as a school leaver and goes all the way to the top of the profession to Level 9, we can all place ourselves within the same Career Framework. But it is not about averaging out the 'scores' on the various Levels. In my role, I am focusing on the Professional Practice Pillar, but I can see that if I was a research assistant, then my Evidence, Research and Development Pillar would be much higher.

Looking at my whole career, not just my current role

I found completing the Career Framework interesting. You are not just looking at the role you are doing now. You can identify with the different Pillars and Levels from previous job roles, because you don't lose the skills that you have gained over the years. I like the idea that you can transfer all your skills into one Career Framework. Even if you don't have those skills acknowledged in your job title, they are making you better at the role you are doing. It is important for me to acknowledge that I haven't lost those skills as I am using them to make my decisions daily. It is great to have that recognised.

Using the Career Framework can help you articulate and demonstrate the skills you have. There are going to be strengths and areas to develop within everyone's profile. If skills haven't been developed yet, it can act as a motivator to learn something new. I like how I can gauge where I am currently and see how I can progress. This would help me develop in my current role, but I can also see how it might help if someone was looking to change roles. You could see what was required for that role, such as leadership responsibilities, and focus on developing in the Leadership Pillar.

For me it is important that the Career Framework is the same for England, Wales, Scotland and Northern Ireland, so whatever you do it is transferable to other settings and areas. We don't appreciate how much we transfer from other roles into our current workplaces. It is nice to see it mapped out on a scale so you can see where you are.

Take-home message

The Career Framework has made me think a lot about how to go forward. It is inspiring to see what I would need to do to get up to the next Level. It has made me look at my current learning in a new way and it will help me to fill in some of the gaps in my current profile. It gives you motivation to further improve.

The Career Framework also helped me to appreciate that what I have learnt and experienced in previous roles is really helping me do my job now. This makes me feel like I have got these skills and I should be using them to their full ability. That was an eye-opener, that I was still using all those skills and they are relevant for occupational therapy.

Examples from the profession

Dr Patricia McClure

EdD, MEd, PGDipEd, PGCUT, BSc Hons, DipCOT, MRCOT, SFHEA, FCHERP

Associate Head of School, School of Health Sciences – Ulster University and Chair of Council – Royal College of Occupational Therapists

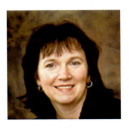

Profile as mapped to the Career Framework:	
■ Professional Practice	8
■ Facilitation of Learning	9
■ Leadership	9
■ Evidence, Research and Development	7

Background

I qualified as an occupational therapist in 1983 and I have thoroughly enjoyed my career in occupational therapy. I practised in mental health services at senior and head levels for 12 years before taking up an academic post in occupational therapy at Ulster University. During that time, I have held the roles of Professional Practice Placement Co-ordinator and Academic Co-ordinator (Professional Lead) for Occupational Therapy and in September 2005, I was appointed as the Associate Head of the School of Health Sciences. I have been actively engaged with the Royal College of Occupational Therapists for many years through a wide range of roles, serving on Council as well as several professional boards, committees and steering groups. I am honoured to have been the Chair of Council of the Royal College of Occupational Therapists since 2015.

My career profile

I guess my strongest Pillars are in Facilitation of Learning and Leadership. I was thinking at first that I was at Level 8 in each of these areas. There appear to be only subtle differences between Levels 8 and 9 and I like leaving room for further development! After a discussion, however, possibly my roles in the university and as Chair of Council for the Royal College of Occupational Therapists could justify me being at Level 9. I imagine that there is still room for development within each Level.

I put myself at a Level 7 for Evidence, Research and Development because in my role I supervise MSc and PhD students, but I don't currently get much time to do hands-on research myself due to the responsibilities of my role as Associate Head of School. It would be great to build up this Pillar, but realistically, there are only so many hours in the day and only so much you can do. I am happy now to be facilitating others to do research, but that won't necessarily show up on my own Pillar!

The Career Framework within university programmes

The Career Framework could be used at all levels of the profession from school leaver, support worker and student to highly experienced people. When occupational therapy students enter their university course (or even before if they are interested in occupational therapy as a career), they could map themselves into the Career Framework. This will help them recognise and value any previous work and voluntary experiences they have gained.

It would be interesting to see how students develop over the duration of their course. That would be a nice research study! In their final year, students could think about their employability and how to prepare for their first position, while also considering where they see themselves going in the future. The Career Framework would enable students and occupational therapists to be more strategic in planning their professional development activities and think about their future career pathway.

At Ulster University, this is an opportune time for us to integrate the Career Framework into our undergraduate programme as we are revalidating the course next year. It will be another useful document on the table for consideration in our curriculum planning preparations.

Using the Career Framework to be bold in our profession

The thing I struggled with when completing my Career Profile was the idea of being '**most** advanced' in Levels 8 and 9. It is interesting that the term 'most advanced' and the other descriptors in the Levels, have come from the European Qualifications Framework. I didn't initially realise that. If these words are being used at a European level, then I can see the value of us thinking about ourselves in these terms.

Occupational therapists often undersell themselves. I think we have an issue with the idea of 'most advanced' as we tend to think 'I am sure there must be someone better'. I have noticed this in discussions with others when asked, for example, to take on a new role or apply for a leadership position and people will often say, "I am sure there is someone better than me to do this?" When asked, "who?", it makes you sit back and reflect, well actually I am as good as anyone else; I do have the right experience and I have a lot to offer.

This is something that we must overcome and change. We need to stop underselling ourselves and acknowledge our skills and expertise. That is where the Career Framework will be useful. In my experience, allied health professionals often become stifled in their career as they are working within structures which limit them from being in the most senior leadership and management positions within health and social care services, as certain positions have historically been restricted to particular professions. Having this Career Framework and using the terms such as 'most advanced' will help us to prove to ourselves, and more importantly to others, that we should be at those most senior levels, in our own right.

Our profession is continuing to grow and develop in confidence. If the Career Framework is used in supervision and appraisals it will really help people to continually reflect on what they are doing, the ways they are working, roles they have and expertise they are developing. It helpfully gives us the words to clearly articulate what we can do, the skills we have and our specialist knowledge and expertise. So, if there is a personnel specification for a job, we will be able to confidently say how we meet the requirements for that role.

Examples from the profession

Let's not get stuck on writing endless different frameworks and competencies

This is *the* Career Framework for occupational therapy. When I looked at the four Pillars and nine Levels within each Pillar, I thought the Career Framework was very comprehensive. The way it considers the overarching principles means it is applicable across the wide range of roles, settings and countries where occupational therapy personnel work. It is important that The Royal College of Occupational Therapists, as our professional body, has developed a Career Framework which is for all four nations of the United Kingdom. It is great that we don't need to 'reinvent the wheel'. I am not aware of such a comprehensive occupational therapy career framework having been developed before.

There appears to be a range of areas where competency frameworks are being developed. When you go down the road of competencies, if you think of all the things an occupational therapist would do within their daily job, there are just so many things. Where do you begin and end? Some competency frameworks can become very cumbersome tools and the potential time spent discussing competencies at all the different levels would be phenomenal. I think these guiding principles are much more user friendly.

Take-home message

The Career Framework is comprehensive. I think it is a great piece of work and the more people use it, the more potential it will have. It is useful to have the conversation with a respected colleague/mentor because you need that sounding board to tease out where you are in the Pillars. The best thing we can do is to start a conversation within the profession about what we are doing in different areas. We need to be comfortable and confident in voicing our skills and abilities. We can all help each other to acknowledge what we are good at and the next steps for our learning and development.

3 What next?

The Career Framework will evolve through a process of continuous evaluation and updates to remain contemporary for the profession. It is important that future work seeks to assess and understand the implementation of the Career Framework and its impact on and for the occupational therapy profession. The future relevance and success of this Career Framework will require on-going co-development with those who use it.

We would value hearing about how you use the Career Framework in practice and would like to keep in touch. Please share your thoughts at: *www.rcot.co.uk* or *https://www.facebook.com/theRCOT* or *www.twitter.com/theRCOT* using #RCOTCareerFramework

Further reading

UK National Occupational Standards (NOS: *http://www.ukstandards.org.uk/Pages/index.aspx*). Accessed on: 14.07.2017.

College of Occupational Therapists (2017) *Professional standards for occupational therapy practice*. London: COT.

College of Occupational Therapists (2015) *Code of ethics and professional conduct*. London: COT.

College of Occupational Therapists (2014) *College of Occupational Therapists' Learning and development standards for pre-registration education*. London: COT.

Top tips for using the Career Framework

- ✔ *Look at all four Pillars of Practice and don't just focus on one or two as they all interlink.* Every role will have elements of all four Pillars, but the Levels are likely to differ.

- ✔ *It is likely that you will be at different Levels across the four Pillars.* This will help you identify potential areas for development as you plan your career. This means your career profile will shift up and down at different points in your working life.

- ✔ *Be brave!* Any self-evaluation can feel daunting or exposing. Working through it, perhaps with a critical friend or trusted peer, can make the process thought-provoking, interesting and enlightening.

- ✔ *Think about yourself and all the experiences, skills and knowledge* acquired throughout your working life, including previous careers. Don't rate yourself according to the confines of your current post – this Career Framework is about you and your own, whole career development.

- ✔ *You do not need to 'tick off' all the guiding principles in a given Level to 'pass' it.* When mapping yourself into the Career Framework, make an intuitive decision on where you feel you best fit according to each Pillar – there is no set formula that needs to be applied.

- ✔ *Appreciate that there is subjectivity in some of the terms.* For example, what do 'most advanced and specialist skills' look like? It is a challenge to think about this in relation to your own area of work, but it can form a basis for discussion. It allows for

What next?

continued growth no matter where you are in your career.

✔ *Think about the Career Framework in your own context.* Debate and discuss it with your colleagues to spark ideas about how it can be used.

✔ *Use the Career Framework flexibly.* Engage with it to discover its many possible uses.

✔ *Don't forget to look at the detailed Guiding Principles avaliable at www.rcot.co.uk.* RCOT members can also access a range of implementation resources.